PMS Clinic
for Women and Girls

PMS Clinic
for Women and Girls

Bonnie Lee

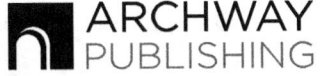
ARCHWAY
PUBLISHING

Archway Publishing books may be ordered through booksellers or by contacting:

Archway Publishing
1663 Liberty Drive
Bloomington, IN 47403
www.archwaypublishing.com
1-(888)-242-5904

Because of the dynamic nature of the Internet, any web addresses or links contained in this book may have changed since publication and may no longer be valid. The views expressed in this work are solely those of the author and do not necessarily reflect the views of the publisher, and the publisher hereby disclaims any responsibility for them.

You should not undertake any diet/exercise regimen recommended in this book before consulting your personal physician. Neither the author nor the publisher shall be responsible or liable for any loss or damage allegedly arising as a consequence of your use or application of any information or suggestions contained in this book.

Any people depicted in stock imagery provided by Thinkstock are models, and such images are being used for illustrative purposes only.
Certain stock imagery © Thinkstock.

ISBN: 978-1-4808-0786-0 (sc)
ISBN: 978-1-4808-0787-7 (e)

Library of Congress Control Number: 2014908815

Printed in the United States of America

Archway Publishing rev. date: 6/17/2014

Dedication

This book is dedicated to all the women and girls who have suffered with premenstrual syndrome, commonly known as *PMS*, enduring high levels of pain and discomfort with inadequate means of relief. It is my hope that my advice and suggestions will help women and girls change the way they feel every day, by making simple nutritional food and beverage changes. By doing so, they will be provided with noticeable relief from all the physical, mental, and emotional pain they have been forced to suffer because of PMS.

Contents

There Is Hope for Eliminating PMS from Your Life!

This book was written for every woman and girl seeking relief from the mental, physical, and emotional pain experienced from premenstrual syndrome. Commonly abbreviated as *PMS*, premenstrual syndrome mimics flu-like symptoms that fall in conjunction with a woman's menstrual cycle. Just the mention of PMS stirs feelings of fear and anxiety in the hearts and minds of women who anticipate experiencing the symptoms. You are probably suffering several types of body aches as well as emotional pain: stiff and sore neck and shoulder muscles, throbbing headaches, emotional distress, sadness, irritability, and frustration. Every month, you anticipate with great anxiety the days you will be forced to endure this terrible pain, which will seem endless!

For the most part, the pain you are experiencing is difficult to relieve, regardless of the brand or amount of pain reliever you use. You are probably bloated and uncomfortable, feeling as though you have gained twenty pounds overnight, not to mention the gut-wrenching cramps. You have tried every pain-relief medication your local drugstores carry, hoping to relieve the pain of headaches, cramps, and general aches, but nothing really works adequately. Your breasts are probably swollen and sore, causing discomfort whether you are wearing a bra or not. When you are wearing a bra, it fits too tightly and is uncomfortable, and you are sure you could burst out of it at any minute. Unfortunately, most medications do not adequately relieve the water retention in your body. As if all this pain wasn't enough to ruin your day and disposition, you are probably also feeling emotionally restless, sad, irritable, and angry. There are days and nights when you struggle in bed or on your couch to find a comfortable position, but your agony is endless. When your pain is at its worst, leaving you feeling helpless and hopeless, you wonder in your despair how it's possible that medical science hasn't yet discovered a medication that will relieve PMS.

When I was suffering with PMS, I remember thinking that I would have been willing to do anything, truly anything, to feel relief from all this terrible pain. Women have stayed in bed anguished and exhausted during a particularly difficult day, worried that they will have an equally painful night as well. They wonder how they will get up in the morning after a bad night to go to their job and do a competent day's work, knowing their job performance, important projects, and meetings will likely be affected in negative ways. This same dread and anxiety also affects planned personal activities that promise to be fun and entertaining. Sometimes the fun has to be cancelled or not planned at all because of PMS pain. You worry you may not be able to participate in activities, risking disappointing family and friends as a no-show, possibly ruining everyone's plans. Many women go to sleep at night feeling perfectly fine and optimistic, just to wake up in the morning to PMS symptoms, which can change or force cancellation of professional and personal plans.

This is the "curse" we always heard about from our mothers and grandmothers when we were growing up. Why have so many of us been condemned to feel so badly every month? Is PMS the price women pay for the gift of childbirth? PMS sufferers ask friends and family for useful advice in dealing with PMS, but aside from suggesting pain medications, they lack helpful options, or like you, they have no idea how to cope. I have no doubt that other women who suffer from PMS would also be willing to try anything to be free of these symptoms, if they only knew how.

Fortunately, I have discovered ways to greatly reduce, and in most cases eliminate, PMS from your life, and the methods are surprisingly simple. I have wonderful, easy-to-implement solutions for you that will make you feel great again, all the time. Now it is time to take those simple, important steps to eliminate the physical, mental, and emotional discomforts of PMS, and return to feeling the way you did before menstrual changes disrupted your life. It is time to restore mental, physical, and emotional comfort for a feeling of health and well-being. There is definitely hope. I offer steps you can take to relieve all this discomfort and return to feeling whole and well again, able to plan and live your life without the pain and inconvenience of PMS. I have written this book to show you how to eliminate PMS, based on my very difficult experiences, and how I learned to prevent and eliminate the symptoms. Doing so finally gave me back the normal, pain-free life I enjoyed prior to the onset of PMS. I know that PMS causes minimal to extreme overall pain for women and girls, making life very difficult to manage physically, mentally, and emotionally. Most of us have heard horror stories from women we have known about PMS symptoms, suffering, and failure to find sufficient relief.

Historically, physicians have had little advice to offer in terms of helping women successfully cope with PMS. Physicians usually recommend diuretics, pain relievers, and hormone therapy, but none of these ever improved the way I felt, or any other women I knew who were suffering from PMS. In fairness to physicians, PMS is a problematic female medical mystery and is difficult to treat. But I have discovered that physicians could help their patients a lot more by advising them to eat foods and beverages low in salt/sodium, sugar, and fat, as well as switching to low-salt/sodium seasonings, which will improve the way women and girls feel in no time. The scientific term for salt is sodium, and appears on all the back labels of food and beverage products, so going forward in this book, I will use the term sodium when discussing salt. For some reason, physicians do not seem to consider the affects sodium, sugar, and fat have on their female patients, nor how to advise them as to more effective means of relief. As many women realize, most pain medications, hormone therapies, and diuretics do not provide enough relief to make very much difference in improving the way they feel. There is also very little helpful published information about PMS, only the usual advertisements promoting hormone treatments and vitamin supplements, none of which are sufficiently helpful. Far too many women and girls have spent their days and nights feeling like they have a bad case of the flu because of PMS, and would be willing to do anything just to feel reasonably normal again. Well, there are ways to feel normal again—in fact, you can feel great all the time! Read on to find out how!

Eliminate PMS by Reducing Sodium, Sugar, and Fat in Food

This is very exciting news for you. You are about to discover how reducing sodium, sugar, and fat in your food and beverages can make you feel terrific again! You'll still be eating and enjoying flavorful foods while discovering why this change is great for you. I believe I can provide solutions that will relieve PMS symptoms without hormonal treatments or expensive vitamin supplements, commonly suggested by physicians and health care professionals. My low sodium, sugar, and fat eating plan will reduce, and in most cases, eliminate PMS from your life. You will not be eating boring food because you will simply be reducing sodium in your diet, not eliminating it. This small change will have you feeling great in no time, and will reduce your anxiety about eating poorly. By making these changes in your food and beverages, you will feel wonderful instead of sick, unmotivated, and bored! With these small adjustments, you will soon be feeling great!

I spent years experimenting with foods, eating all types prepared in different ways, trying to determine which recipes tasted best to me, and at the same time, I wanted to be healthy and eliminate PMS.

I rarely ate junk foods; neither did my friends. For years, my friends and I thought we were eating well-balanced diets that would make us feel great and keep us healthy. Strangely enough, in spite of all our efforts, we weren't feeling that well before or during our periods, and we couldn't understand why. We didn't realize we weren't recognizing the mistakes we were making in terms of food purchases and how we were preparing and seasoning our meals. There were flaws in the ingredients contained in the foods and beverages we were consuming, regardless of whether they were bought at fast-food restaurants or prepared at home. I discovered I was making some serious mistakes by consuming foods and beverages that contained too much sodium, sugar, and fat.

My biggest concern became sodium because in researching it, I discovered how adversely it affects the body, causing swelling, general aches, tenderness, irritability and severe headaches, which is PMS. Sodium causes these symptoms because it increases fluid retention in the body. This led me to read the ingredient labels on all food products in the grocery store, which was the most important step I could make. I learned that most of the food I was buying was high in sodium, sugar, and fat, and these ingredients really were affecting me in negative ways. Until I became aware of the harm I was doing to myself by eating too much of these ingredients, I thought I was eating healthy, flavorful foods, and assumed I was preparing everything in a healthy and delicious manner. By experimenting with foods and seasonings in general, I discovered I needed to eliminate a lot of processed (packaged) food products because of the high levels of sodium, sugar, and fat, which were causing elevated PMS symptoms. I also realized I had to learn to stop adding too much of these ingredients in my conventional home cooking.

I learned that I had to stop purchasing many food items, and noticed other women were making bad food purchases as well. The problem with most processed foods is that these products contain high levels of sodium, sugar, and fat, which cause PMS. So the best way you can protect yourself against PMS is by not consuming them. If you want to feel better quickly, it is time to eliminate processed foods, purchase the freshest foods possible, and change the seasonings you use when preparing them. Heathcare professionals regularly provide guidance to the public that sodium reduction is important to maintain good health. Taking these steps will undoubtedly make all the difference in the world in how you feel. It made sense to me, and by following these guidelines, I finally became pain free and felt great!

Wow! This was so exciting! I was anxious to leave my old negative eating habits behind as soon as possible. Although I would miss eating some food favorites I had enjoyed for years, it would be worth abandoning them to live without pain. Feeling better was worth much more to me than clinging to old favorites that were making me feel miserable. Relief from PMS pain was worth more than words could express. No more pain! I would gladly stop eating poor food choices immediately to feel great and like my old self again. I had discovered what I believed was a miracle—that I could feel great again every day, simply by eating differently. You cannot ignore the positive benefits of how great you will feel and the general feeling of well-being you will get simply by reducing your intake of sodium, sugar, and fat. Now that I knew how to eliminate PMS, all I had to do was head to the grocery store and shop in a different way, making smarter food and beverage choices. Making these food choices became easy for me and will be easy for you as well when you realize how great you feel almost immediately. Preparing fresh, healthy foods, and seasoning in a low-sodium manner will be a new experience for you, but making these changes to be healthier and free from PMS symptoms should be exciting for you. Of course you want to feel better, and you deserve to, so let the changes begin! Say good-bye to negative old eating habits, and look forward to enjoying how great you will feel, and your increased sense of well-being. By changing the way you choose foods, seasonings, beverages, and desserts, you can change the way you feel to that of healthy and great! So now is the time for you to begin a new adventure and start on your journey to a happy life of feeling great!

Smart Food and Seasoning Choices

Everyone knows it is smart to eat in a healthy manner, but for those who suffer from PMS, it is essential to limit the amounts of sodium, sugar, and fat to feel good. You have probably noticed that the only people who seem to take dietary recommendations seriously are those with life-threatening medical conditions, whose physicians bluntly tell them that their lives depend on changing their diets. PMS is not considered a life-threatening condition; however, for women who have PMS, it is a threat to their health, well-being, and ability to live a normal life. Sustaining a healthy, pain-free lifestyle if you suffer from PMS requires reductions in sodium, sugar, and fat. During stressful days, it is very easy to consume too much of these. When we are stressed, we do not think rationally, and usually reach for junk food to ease our anxiety, with no thought to how we will feel later in the day, tomorrow, or in a week. This causes a negative repetitive cycle, because when our stress disappears and we are calmer, we realize our actions will likely cause PMS, which leads to more stress, anxiety and more PMS pain. You wish you could turn back the clock and make better choices, and you wonder how you could have treated yourself so poorly, making matters worse.

The best method by which to change how you react to stress or boredom is to keep snacks, food, and beverages handy that taste good, but pose no threat of triggering PMS symptoms. This means they must be low in sodium, sugar, and fat, so your body will not react negatively to stress or experience PMS. By keeping these types of foods easily accessible, you will not be as inclined to reach for salty, sugar-laden junk food during stressful times. Positive, healthy eating habits will modify your knee-jerk reaction to crave and reach for junk food. Begin now by keeping healthy snacks and beverages nearby to satisfy your needs.

Because you are ready to start new eating habits, you can look forward to making exciting life style plans, which will be uninterrupted by PMS symptoms. I am about to tell you more about how to do it. This is an exciting time for you because you have made the decision to eat and enjoy beverages differently, so that you can change your life in wonderful ways you can only imagine!

Begin by making a trip to the grocery store, so that you can load up on fresh food and low-salt and no-salt-added seasonings to flavor your food. You will be making simple, delicious meals that will have you feeling great in no time at all! Keep in mind, your taste buds will be adjusting to the reduced sodium you are now using, so give yourself a chance to adapt to your new way of seasoning food. Also remember that while making these changes, you should avoid fast food if at all possible. Fast-food tastes good and is quick and convenient, but it is loaded with high levels of sodium, sugar, and sometimes unhealthy amounts of fat. Most oils are healthy to consume, however, it is wise to limit red meat fats from your diet, because these build hormones in the body that cause breast tenderness and fluid retention. Eating too much red meat fat is your enemy, because it triggers PMS. Remember, you are making a commitment to be kind to yourself by staying away from fast food and other poor food options. Focus on choices that will make you feel good. You will be getting your life back by doing so.

Fresh fruits and vegetables are important in eliminating PMS. Many people are often scared off by the prices of fresh fruits and vegetables at the grocery store, so begin by purchasing the more reasonably priced items. Be alert when purchasing conventional canned or frozen fruits and vegetables, since those usually contain higher sodium and sugar contents. A trick you can use if you prefer the lower prices and convenience of canned fruits and vegetables is to open the can, drain the fluid, and rinse the fruits or vegetables with water. This is an extra step you need to take to eliminate the sodium and sugary fluids. After you have done this, add your own low-salt seasonings or no-sugar-added sweetener.

A great way to purchase fresh fruits and vegetables is by going to discount grocery stores for lower prices. Discount stores provide a wide variety of fresh fruits, vegetables, entrées, desserts, and seasonings. You should purchase garlic, onion, and low-salt or no-salt seasonings, as well as olive oil, since they are the healthiest choices you can make to season your food and guard against PMS.

Another important habit you will begin implementing is reading the back labels on everything that interests you at the grocery store before you make a purchase. You will develop a keen awareness of ingredient labelling on all products, since you will be paying close attention to the milligrams (ml/mg) of sodium, sugar, and fat contained in all products. Doing so is crucial to reducing PMS and feeling great again. Sodium is probably your worst enemy, and eating as little sodium as possible is very important in eliminating headaches, uncomfortable swelling, bloating, stiff neck, shoulder muscles, and other discomforts.

The best seasonings to use in foods are fresh onion and garlic, found in the produce section of grocery stores. Onion powder and garlic powder are wonderful seasonings for food, not to mention convenient, and can be found in the seasonings/baking aisle of the grocery store. <u>Do not use garlic salt</u>, which can be confused with garlic powder, since this is another form of sodium, and must be avoided. Just make sure you are choosing products that are very low in sodium, or you will be defeating the purpose of preparing low-sodium food and beverages. Seasonings have really evolved, and there are many spices on market shelves that can be used to flavor food very well that contain little or no sodium, so simply look at the back labels to be sure. Since you are accustomed to using salt, it may take a little while for your taste buds to adjust to a more reduced salt flavor. Should this be a problem for you initially, try using tiny amounts of salt or salt substitutes that will provide some salt flavor. Over use of salt not only causes severe PMS symptoms, but contributes to other serious medical conditions, such as high blood pressure and diabetes.

I have noticed that using very little salt over the years to eliminate PMS has been a blessing in disguise, because doing so has prevented me from developing common medical conditions. My physician gives me high marks for being in excellent health, requiring no medications. So the less sodium, sugar and fat you use, the better you will feel, and the healthier you will be for a variety of reasons.

Another good idea for flavoring your food is experimenting with herbs, since they are very flavorful and do not contain sodium, sugar and fat. They add great flavor and pizzazz to a wide variety of foods, so have some fun and experiment. Herbs can be purchased at grocery stores in the spice and produce sections, and if you really enjoy them, you can plant an herb garden at home, so you can conveniently pick and choose appropriate herbs just outside your door for your meals. You could be developing a new fun satisfying hobby, while at the same time improving your health. Herb gardens require little space, and are easy to grow in ordinary soil. As we all know, home-grown food always tastes better and is healthier for you too, so give it a try!

While grocery shopping, consider switching to healthier, low-sodium cooking oils and margarine spreads as well. Some margarines and oils contain elevated sodium levels and are unhealthy fats. It is easy to overlook some of the negative characteristics in certain cooking oils, butter, margarine, shortening, and lard, because you've been using them for years without giving it a second thought. They are the invisible offenders with elevated sodium levels, and can be harmful to PMS sufferers, so I recommend using olive oil and margarines with low sodium levels instead. Extra virgin olive oil is particularly excellent for cooking and making tasty salad dressings and marinades. Healthcare professionals recommend it because it is rich in monounsaturated fats, which reduce unhealthy cholesterol, and boost healthy cholesterol. It is also exceptionally healthy because it is mechanically processed, which means antioxidents called polyphenols mop up free radicals before causing damage to arteries. Like most people, you have probably used traditional types of oils over the years, which are fine. Chefs recommend using olive oil because it has a nice, mild flavor that complements food, whether cooked or not. It is also more digestible than other types of oils, so you most likely will not experience indigestion and irregularity. Try mixing up some olive oil and vinegar, and add some great packaged or fresh herbs that are low in sodium. Save time on chopping garlic by using shortcuts like purchasing bottled chopped garlic, and try adding chopped cilantro, green onion and other herbs for great taste. I love it, and I bet you will too!

As you change the way you prepare food, you will find it easy to reduce sodium, sugar, and fat in recipes you normally use. Doing so will become a habit, and it is really very easy, since you will only be making moderate changes. You will find you feel better with each passing day. Sometimes you have hectic days that leave little time to cook and prepare meals, so go ahead and pick out a low sodium, sugar, and fat meal and dessert from the frozen section of your grocery store. Frozen food manufacturers recognize that their customers have become more health conscious, so frozen food has really evolved, providing you with healthy, tasty choices that are low in sodium, sugar, and fat that you will enjoy. After you have finished your meal, it is time for dessert, and you will find the frozen and diet sections of your grocery stores carry reduced-sugar and no-sugar-added desserts of all types that you will find delicious. So you see, you will not feel deprived, but will continue to enjoy tasty meals and delicious desserts, knowing you are doing the very best for yourself!

Checking Food Labels for Sodium, Sugar, and Fat

PMS symptoms include headaches, water retention, an uncomfortable bloated body, irritability and general aches and pains. All these symptoms are caused by consuming too much sodium, sugar and fat. I have explained that eliminating PMS sympstoms starts by following a healthier diet plan that is as low in sodium, sugar and fat as possible. You are probably wondering how to go about doing this, and wonder how you will know what is considered low and appropriate for a PMS sufferer? Begin by purchasing foods and beverages that contain as little sodium, sugar and fat as possible. You will become familar with the ingredient listings on the back labels of grocery products. Junk food contains astronomical amounts of sodium, sugar and fat, which will give you a very bad case of PMS, so I recommend not making these purchases. In planning your meals and snacks, choose those with back labels listing the lowest levels of sodium, sugar and fat as possible. You are about to become an expert in paying close attention to the milligrams/milliliters of sodium, sugar, and fat contained in food products, because it is very important that you eat as little as possible of these ingredients to feel well. In addition, you will be paying close attention to the serving size listed on the back label. Milligrams/milliliters, commonly known as ml/mg, and serving size are very important and closely linked to each other because they determine how much product is safe for you to consume. On the next page, I have provided an example of how a typical back label of an average canned product looks, and how the ingredients are listed. Most canned/processed food products contain more sodium, sugar, and fat than you can tolerate as a PMS sufferer, and you are probably eating many of these products right now, which is the reason you have PMS. You should eliminate these products immediately to begin feeling well. The serving sizes and ingredient listings vary with food and beverage companies. Companies frequently change their labels, as well as the manner in which they list their ingredients and serving sizes, so this can be a little confusing to consumers trying to make good healthy decisions about which foods and beverages they should purchase. Stay focused on the ml/mg listings of sodium, sugar, and fat amounts contained in the serving size, which is usually shown as 1/2 cup to 1 cup. Check to see how many ml of sodium, sugar and fat are in a serving size, and that will tell you how much of the product you can eat to avoid PMS symptoms. Many product serving sizes simply contain too much sodium, sugar and fat for you to tolerate, putting you at risk to suffer severe PMS headaches and other discomforts. It is very important to be aware of this information, so that you limit the amounts you eat to feel well. Just remember, sodium, sugar, and fat are "the evil three," because they are responsible for your PMS suffering every month, making your life anything but heavenly, so eat them sparingly.

At this point, you are just becoming familiar with the product back labels and the content information listed, so I will go into more detail to make it clearer which products contain the least amounts of sodium, sugar and fat. I have provided an example of a typical product label. It may look complicated, but if you look closely, you will become familiar with the nutritional information listed, as well as the mg/ml of sodium, sugar and fat contained in the product. Your goal is to purchase products with the least amount of sodium, sugar, and fat, so that you reduce your chances of experiencing PMS. The back product label example shown is of a canned product containing typically high amounts of sodium, that most people would purchase for flavor enjoyment and relieve hunger. For a PMS sufferer, however, this product would most likely cause horrific PMS symptoms, because of the high levels of sodium.

Nutritional Facts

Serving Size 1 cup (240 mL)
Servings per Container about 2
Amount per Serving
Calories 210
Calories from Fat 90

Total Fat 10g
Saturated Fat 1.5g
Trans Fat 0g
Cholesterol 5mg
Sodium 890mg
Total Carbohydrate 23g

Dietary Fiber 3g

Sugars 1g

Protein 6g

Vitamin A (Trivial ingredients listed on labels)

Vitamin C (Trivial ingredients listed on labels)

Several nutritional ingredients are shown, but the one that will put you at PMS risk is the high sodium mg number. This ingredient has the potential to be the most harmful to you in causing PMS. The sodium, fat, and sugar mL/mg numbers will always be the numbers to check on all product labels for the reasons I have explained. The lower the mL/mg numbers, the better, making you less likely to suffer with PMS. These three ingredients are causing your PMS, and if you have severe PMS, can be even more harmful, even if eaten in small quantities. The sodium number listed of 890 ml is high, so it shouldn't be eaten by someone who easily experiences severe headaches, aches and pain, because it will cause PMS. Remember, consumption of sodium, sugar and fat causes the body to retain fluid, causing bloating, breast tenderness, irritability, sadness and headaches. The sugar and fat mg levels in this product are very low, so they would generally be safe to eat. However, since the sodium number is so high, it is very likely that this product will cause a PMS headache. Remember, the rule to follow, is that for anything you are considering eating, make sure it contains the lowest possible sodium, sugar, and fat, therefore reducing your chances of triggering PMS symptoms. As an additional helpful guide, I have listed the amounts of sodium, sugar, and fat that would be safe for you to eat at every meal, helping you to avoid PMS. I arrived at these numbers based on my research, my experience, and that of other women and girls, who reduced their sodium, sugar and fat consumption, and therefore were able to greatly reduce and eliminate PMS. These guidelines are safe for anyone to use, regardless of ethnicity, age, or lifestyle. Healthcare professionals strongly advise their patients, and Americans in general, to reduce their sodium, sugar and fat consumption, so they will be healthier. These guidelines can help prevent heart disease, obesity, and a myriad of health conditions. Reductions in sodium, sugar and fat reduced PMS symptoms for me, as well as other women and girls, and can do the same for you! You may want to check with your physician for their recommendations, but these are safe effective guidelines.

❖ The *sodium* levels should be between 500 and 700 mL/mg *per meal*.

❖ The *fat* levels should be about 15 mL/mg *per meal*.

❖ The *sugar* levels should be about 15 mL/mg *per meal*.

It becomes easy to check labels on food packages for levels of sodium, sugar, and fat. You will become quite good at recognizing the products that pose no PMS threat, as well as avoiding those that do. In choosing your food and beverages, you will also be experimenting to find the best sodium, sugar and fat levels for you—levels that provide enough flavor in your food and beverages, without causing PMS pain. Also remember that your taste buds will be adapting to these lower ingredient levels, so be patient. Although the levels I have listed may seem low, you will feel significantly better for making these small changes, and you will find that eating lower levels of sodium, sugar, and fat will be well worth doing because you will feel so great!

I have provided another product back label example that contains ingredients that would be safe to consume. These will not likely cause PMS, because of the low sodium, sugar, and fat levels. This product contains levels that are safe and acceptable.

Nutritional Facts

Serving Size 1 cup (243g)

Servings per Container about 2

Amount per Serving

Calories 90

Calories from Fat 10

Total Fat 1g

Saturated Fat 0g

Trans Fat 0g

Cholesterol 15mg

Total Carbohydrate 12g

Dietary Fiber 1g

Sugars 2g

Protein 8g

Sodium 390mg

Take a look at the difference in sodium levels of the two product labels I have provided. The comparisons are striking. The difference in sodium levels is a whopping 500 milligrams. So, to avoid PMS symptoms, you should choose the product with only 390 milligrams of sodium, which also has low sugar and fat levels, making it safe for you to eat. Traditional snack and dessert products are known for having very high sodium, sugar, and fat levels. That is why you will need to be selective in the grocery store and pay close attention to the numbers and serving size when making your food and beverage choices, so that you will keep your mg/ml numbers as low as possible. The most positive choice you can make for yourself to be free of PMS is to eat about 1,800 milligrams total per day, or less. This number represents a low daily total food consumption of sodium, sugar and fat, which is ideal to reduce/eliminate PMS symptoms. Most people eat well over 2,000 ml per day, and usually considerably more. 1,800 ml is much lower compared to the usual 2,000+ sodium, sugar and fat intake most people consume daily. Over 2000+ is considered unhealthy by most healthcare professionals, because it means the average person is regularly consuming high levels of sodium, sugar and fat. Based on my research and personal experience, 1,800 ml is appropriate for a low sodium, sugar and fat diet, and is ideal for PMS sufferers, and also provides healthy outcomes for any ethnicity, age, or lifestyle. You are probably accustomed to eating food and beverages that are very salty, sugary, and fattening. A great way to help you adapt to healthier food and beverage consumption, and relieve hunger pangs is by eating more fruits, vegetables, and fresh or raw grains with your meals, or eat them as snacks during your day. These foods contain little, if any sodium, so they are perfect additions to meals and great as snacks. Occasionally, you may exceed eating 1,800 ml per day, but if that happens, simply make further sodium, sugar, and fat reductions in your meals and snacks during the days that follow.

Sometimes your days will be particularly hectic, leaving little time for preparing meals, so purchase ready-made meals at the grocery store, choosing a low-sodium, sugar, and fat meal from the frozen section, but be careful to watch the numbers. Most frozen foods have high sodium, sugar, and fat levels, so be sure to choose the ones that don't. Also check the diet aisles for good choices as well. Some canned and frozen foods with lower sodium levels are available and are also appropriate for you. Remember, you do not have to limit yourself to fresh at all times, but it is preferable. Just watch the levels of sodium, sugar, and fat in the food and beverage items you are considering. Frozen foods are great for meals, snacks, and desserts, so simply check for the lowest numbers. By doing so, you'll be enjoying your life free from PMS in no time at all!

The Joy of Party Food

The whole point of eating dessert is to have something delicious and sweet after your meal. It is easy to eat desserts and snacks because they taste so good, and it is easy to overindulge. Parties and social gatherings inspire us to consume delicious rich foods, decadent desserts, and exotic alcoholic beverages because they are part of the festive atmosphere. Parties and social gatherings draw friends and family together, and promote the attitude of throwing caution to the wind, partying as though there is no tomorrow. After drinking your first cocktail, you convince yourself that sampling a little bit of everything won't hurt. The buffet table is tempting you to indulge with abandon, but try to make good choices, and eat and drink selectively. Eating too much sugar will bring on a variety of PMS discomforts, such as irritability, depression and sadness. Unfortunately, doing so is often quite troublesome to those suffering from PMS, so try to use some restraint and good judgment in what you are consuming. You will thank yourself later when you are feeling well and not combating PMS.

Another reason women and girls eat salty, sugary food is stress. Stress is the trigger that prompts us to eat everything that we shouldn't, such as sugary desserts, salty, fat-laden snacks, sugary beverages, and alcoholic drinks. As wonderful as they taste, they are our enemies, causing serious PMS discomfort because of the high sugar content. Sugar causes the blues, for sure! After indulging, we often experience a letdown, with accompanying feelings of sadness, irritability, anxiety, bloating, and overall negativity. We usually eat sugary foods and beverages when we are emotionally upset and stressed. They are almost impossible to resist when we feel this way. Everyone has heard of the sugar blues, and when it comes to PMS, this is no exaggeration. Eating ordinary sugar causes irritability, sadness, and listlessness, all of which prevent women and girls from feeling well, robbing them of their motivation to engage in all types of activities, and leaving them unable to enjoy life in general.

Dessert companies know very well that most of us have a sweet tooth, so they produce wide varieties of candy and sweets for us to enjoy. However, they have also become aware that many of us require dessert and snack alternatives for health reasons, so they have formulated new products to satisfy our need for sweets in a healthier way. Food companies realize their customers have become much more health conscious, and aware of how detrimental sugar is to good health. Fortunately, manufacturers have made it possible for us to enjoy desserts, snacks, and beverages that are lower in sugar and fat by using sugar substitutes in their products. Fortunately, as consumers, there are many sugar substitute products available in most grocery stores that are very tasty, and very close to sugar flavor. Perhaps you enjoy fruit snacks and desserts. Head for the frozen section, and you will likely find many delicious choices to enjoy.

Perhaps you like baking, so why not try making your own favorite low, or no-sugar desserts and snacks? Keep them on hand whether at home or work, so you can grab them whenever you need a sweet treat. You will be surprised how flavorful they are, and you will enjoy them without feeling guilty, and without the anxiety of eating sugar, which you know will cause PMS. I do this all the time, and it seems like I'm always whipping up my usual desserts and trying new ones by using a sugar substitute instead of real sugar. So, choose food items that are similar to those you normally enjoy by using ingredient substitutions that are as low as possible in sodium, sugar, and fat. That way, you can enjoy them anywhere, anytime, and have great-tasting, quick, and easy desserts readily available. By doing so, you will be less likely to purchase desserts that will cause PMS. So, you see, you have better options than you thought, and all these delicious low sodium, sugar, and fat choices will help keep you from missing out on all the fun of enjoying wonderful desserts!

Tracking Your Food
and Beverages

You may find it helpful to track what you are eating and drinking every day for a month and note how you feel. Assuming you have reduced your sodium, sugar, and fat consumption, you should be feeling better with each passing day. If you find that you do not feel well on a given day, refer back to your tracking sheet to determine what you ate or drank that may have contained too much sodium, sugar, or fat. This will help you determine which foods or drinks you should reduce or eliminate altogether, so that your PMS symptoms will diminish. By tracking for a month the way you feel based on what you eat and drink, you will become aware of what you should eliminate, and what you can continue to consume. On the next two pages, I have set up a monthly grid so that you can make notes and track what you eat and drink and describe how you feel on any given day. By doing so, you will determine which foods and beverages are triggering your PMS symptoms, therefore learning to avoid them. You can make copies of these grids for as many months as you'd like, if that will help you track this information, or make up your own tracking sheets, if that is more helpful.

Monthly Food and Beverage Tracking Sheet

Food and Beverages	PMS Symptoms
1.	
2.	
3.	
4.	
5.	
6.	
7.	
8.	
9.	
10.	
11.	
12.	

13.	
14.	
15.	
16.	
17.	
18.	
19.	
20.	
21.	
22.	
23.	
24.	
25.	
26.	
27.	
28.	

29.	
30.	
31.	

Looking Forward to
Your New Life

Women and girls deserve to wake up every morning feeling great, and it is possible to feel good again by making the simple changes I have described. I have suggested easy ways for women and girls to change their diets, so their lives will no longer be adversely affected by PMS. Most women and girls want to feel assured that they can enjoy their lives, whether they are going to work, school, or participating in other activities without dreading that PMS will ruin their plans for any given day. Women and girls can live wonderful lives uninterrupted, and experience well-being and improved good health, without the anxiety and pain of PMS. PMS is a condition that can be reversed by making the reliable changes in food and beverage consumption that I have described.

Over the years, I have spoken with women and girls suffering from PMS, and they believe this is one of the most important and frustrating health issues they face. They are right, and adopting this new way of eating will undoubtedly be of great value to you, and open up endless possibilities to enjoy the freedom to live happily every day of your life. PMS will not be a problem. This new way of approaching food, beverages, and nutrition will not only make you feel great, but you will lose weight, improve your overall health, and impress your physician with healthier blood test results. This may sound strange, but PMS is a mysterious blessing in disguise, because it forces you to eat better, making you healthier. If you are serious about eliminating PMS from your life and follow the advice in this book, you will be reaping huge health benefits on a long-term basis over the years. You will have lower blood pressure and cholesterol levels, effectively fighting heart disease, and other medical conditions. Chances are you will also not develop diabetes and obesity, which are at epidemic levels, needlessly killing so many Americans every year. This new way of approaching food and nutrition will make you feel great! You will be preparing delicious meals, beverages, and desserts by using ingredients that eliminate PMS. It is in your best interest to follow my advice to eliminate headaches, bloating, irritability, sadness, and general body pain. I am reaching out to you and other women and girls, knowing that all of you can be helped with this problematic medical condition. My intent is to give you hope with the simple changes I have recommended, so you can manage your meals, beverages, and snacks, and improve your lives, which will no longer be at the mercy of PMS.

I imagine most women want to feel assured that they can enjoy their lives, whether at work or play, without dreading that PMS may ruin their plans for the day and their future. PMS is a condition that can be reversed, using reliable nutritional changes and by changing eating habits. Women and girls can lead pain-free lives without limitations. It is time for you, other women, and girls to start a new life with simple nutritional changes. You can live without the burdens that PMS places upon you, so that you can look forward to feeling great, and lead an active, joyful life now, tomorrow, and for the rest of your life!

www.ingramcontent.com/pod-product-compliance
Lightning Source LLC
Chambersburg PA
CBHW060005300526
45794CB00003B/1094